Dog-Kissed Tears

Dog-Kissed Tears

Songs of Friendship, Loss, and Healing

LAMBERT ZUIDERVAART

RESOURCE *Publications* • Eugene, Oregon

DOG-KISSED TEARS
Songs of Friendship, Loss, and Healing

Copyright © 2010 Lambert Zuidervaart. All rights reserved. Except for brief quotations in critical publications or reviews, no part of this book may be reproduced in any manner without prior written permission from the publisher. Write: Permissions, Wipf and Stock Publishers, 199 W. 8th Ave., Suite 3, Eugene, OR 97401.

Resource Publications
An Imprint of Wipf and Stock Publishers
199 W. 8th Ave., Suite 3
Eugene, OR 97401
www.wipfandstock.com

ISBN 13: 978-1-60899-700-8

Manufactured in the U.S.A.

The Scripture quotations contained herein are from the New Revised Standard Version Bible: Catholic Edition, copyright © 1993 and 1989 by the Division of Christian Education of the National Council of the Churches of Christ in the U.S.A. Used by permission. All rights reserved.

The publishers listed have given permission to use quotations from the following copyrighted lyrics.

"Festival of Friends"
Written by Bruce Cockburn
Copyright © 1988 Golden Mountain Music Corp. (SOCAN)
Used by permission.

"Healer of Our Every Ill" by Marty Haugen
Copyright © 1987 by GIA Publications, Inc.,
7404 S. Mason Ave., Chicago, IL 60638
www.giamusic.com 800.442.1358
All rights reserved. Used by permission.

"Fields of Gold"
Music and Lyrics by Sting
© 1993 STEERPIKE LTD.
Administered by EMI MUSIC PUBLISHING LIMITED
All Rights Reserved International Copyright Secured
Used by Permission
Reprinted by permission of Hal Leonard Corporation

"Fragile"
Music and Lyrics by Sting
© 1987 G.M. SUMNER
Administered by EMI MUSIC PUBLISHING LIMITED
All Rights Reserved International Copyright Secured
Used by Permission
Reprinted by permission of Hal Leonard Corporation

"Precious Lord, Take My Hand"
Words and Music by Thomas A. Dorsey
Copyright © 1938 by Unichappell Music Inc.
Copyright Renewed
International Copyright Secured All Rights Reserved
Reprinted by permission of Hal Leonard Corporation

"I'm So Lonesome I Could Cry"
Words and Music by Hank Williams
Copyright © 1949 Sony/ATV Music Publishing LLC and Hiriam Music in the U.S.A.
Copyright Renewed
All Rights on behalf of Hiriam Music Administered by Rightsong Music Inc.
All Rights outside the U.S.A. Administered by Sony/ATV Music Publishing LLC
All Rights on behalf of Sony/ATV Music Publishing LLC
Administered by Sony/ATV Music Publishing LLC, 8 Music Square West, Nashville, TN 37203
International Copyright Secured All Rights Reserved
Reprinted by permission of Hal Leonard Corporation

Photography courtesy of the author.

For Joyce and to the memory of my parents
Thank you for gracing my life.

Contents

1. Prelude: Songs of Benjamin 1
2. Lead Me Home 5
3. Retrieval 11
4. Comfort 15
5. Fragile 19
6. Snow on Snow 25
7. Blessing 29
8. Rest Gently, Gently Rest 33
9. Benediction 39
10. Field of Love 45
11. Healing 49
12. Reunion 53
13. Alone 57
14. Homecoming 61
15. Postlude: Elegy 65

Acknowledgments 69
Notes 75

1

Prelude: Songs of Benjamin

> An elegant song won't hold up long
> When the palace falls and the parlour's gone
> We all must leave but it's not the end
> We'll meet again at the festival of friends.
>
> Smiles and laughter and pleasant times
> There's love in the world but it's hard to find
> I'm so glad I found you—I'd just like to extend
> An invitation to the festival of friends.[1]

I DID not *plan* to write this book. I *needed* to write it. I needed to celebrate the gift of friendship. And I wanted to lament the loss of a friend. The friend is a dog named Rosa. A beautiful Golden Retriever / Labrador Retriever mix whose noble bearing and affectionate ways would melt the stoniest heart, Rosa was my loving companion for fifteen years. Her gentle nudge and waving tail said that she welcomed all visitors both big and small.

Rosa lies at the center of my circle of human friends. I am connected to them through her. When Rosa died in February 2005, this circle drew near. They shared my grief and encouraged my journey without her. This book celebrates their friendship along with hers. Indirectly the book also laments two losses in this intimate circle. Jeanie

Zinkand died at age 47 in August 2000. Esther Hart died at age 39 in April 2007. Jeanie, the mother of our goddaughter Kate; Esther, our own goddaughter, and the mother of a very special little girl named Sophie—both of them cut down by cancer, both of them best friends of my wife Joyce Recker, and my friends too. I do not know how to write directly about losing Jeanie and Esther and about our longing for their companionship. In writing about Rosa, I am also thinking of them.

There have been other losses. One of our friends lost his lover to a sudden heart attack. Two were abruptly and unjustly dismissed from jobs they enjoyed, by an institution they faithfully served. Another friend went through a devastating separation and divorce. Two others have lost both their mother and their best friend to cancer. This book celebrates their friendships with us and laments their losses too.

I think of my meditations on friendship, loss, and healing as "Songs of Benjamin." The title stems from my inspiration to write a poem about friendship. Toni and her friend Cliff were visiting us in Toronto during the summer after Rosa had died. We were reminiscing about the house where Joyce and I had lived before moving to Toronto in 2002. It was a stately Arts and Crafts home in a pleasant neighborhood on Benjamin Avenue in Grand Rapids, Michigan. Joyce had a sun-filled piano studio off the first-floor living room, and I had a grand study on the second floor. My study overlooked a spacious backyard that Joyce had turned into an urban oasis. Both the study and the yard were Rosa's rooms. During our nine years there, the Benjamin house became a hub of hospitality and healing. On the day we left for Toronto, Joyce and I walked through the entire house one last time. Despite our eagerness to move, leaving this lovely home, with all of its good memories, made us very sad.

As we reminisced with Toni and Cliff, I suddenly had the title for an unwritten poem: "Singing a Song of Benjamin." I did not know when I would write the poem, or on what occasion. I only knew it would reflect the years we lived in our favorite home. But my sudden inspiration pointed to more than a poem. A month or so later I began to consider writing meditations about my canine companion. I called them "Walking with Rosa"—a rather pedestrian label! When I began to write them, however, "Songs of Benjamin" became the working title. For while writing I recalled how central the Benjamin house had been to Rosa's life with us. She was three years old when we moved to 315 Benjamin, and we moved to Toronto three years before she died. Our circle of friends had come together at Benjamin.

Right now I imagine Rosa lounging there on the living room rug. Our friends from those years gather around her and sing her songs of Benjamin: Ron, Connie and Darlene, Toni, Daryl and Dan, Randy, Dave and Wendy, Thea, Donna and Bill, Matt, Simona and Will, Clarence, Henry, Marj, Paul, Ruth. Our family members, colleagues, and more recent acquaintances stand nearby. Peering over Joyce's shoulders and mine, and humming lightly, are Jeanie, Esther, and their loved ones. Katie and little Sophie softly stroke our gentle dog. Rosa stretches out on her side. She sighs in bliss, lullabied within a festival of friends.

"Benjamin" is an ambivalent name. According to Hebrew stories, Rachel named her second son "Benoni" or "son of my pain." She had a difficult pregnancy, as did our Jeanie and Esther, and died in childbirth. Rachel's hundred-year-old husband Jacob promptly renamed his twelfth and youngest son "Binjamin" or "son of [my] right." Here "right" means the right-hand side. It might refer to the south—the tribe of Benjamin settled to the south of Ephraim, a more dominant tribe. On a different spelling, the name might refer to Jacob's old age. This "son of the south" or "son of my old age" was Jacob's most cherished child, born to Rachel, his favorite wife. Many years later, Joseph, whose brothers had sold him into slavery, threatened to enslave Benjamin, in order to test their remorse. Just before this test, however, when he first saw Benjamin at an Egyptian state dinner, Joseph, successful slave-turned-ruler, was moved to tears.

My songs of Benjamin retain this ambivalence. Like Rachel, I do not wish to hide the pain that accompanies their birth. They are songs of loss and longing. Yet the sorrow to which they give voice is sung through tears of joy. They are tears of gratitude for the healing Rosa, our faithful retriever, carried into my life, even as I shed them in sadness over her departure. I write in order to thank her for the smiles and laughter and pleasant times—the love in the world she helped me find. I'm so glad we found her. She so liked to extend her invitation to our festival of friends.

2

Lead Me Home

> Precious Lord, take my hand
> Lead me on, let me stand
> I am tired, I am weak, I am worn;
> Through the storm, through the night,
> Lead me on to the light:
>
> Take my hand, precious Lord,
> Lead me home.
>
> When the darkness appears
> And the night draws near
> And the day is past and gone,
> At the river I stand,
> Guide my feet, hold my hand:
>
> Take my hand, precious Lord,
> Lead me home.[2]

JOYCE AND I were driving back to Grand Rapids one weekend in April 1990 when I popped the question about adopting a dog. We had been in Ann Arbor for the day to celebrate the decision by MIT Press to publish *Adorno's Aesthetic Theory*, my first academic book. I had been working on it since Joyce and I were married thirteen years before.

It had been more than twenty years since I last had a dog. During those years I had lived in many places: Iowa, Toronto, Berlin, Amsterdam, Edmonton. The five most recent years, at our first house in Grand Rapids, were the longest either of us had stayed in one place since leaving our parental homes. We would be staying longer. Now seemed a better time than ever before to welcome a dog into our lives.

Still tentative and unsure, we visited the Humane Society of Kent County the next weekend. The kennels were full. Dogs of many ages and types watched as we walked and talked: old timers and plump puppies, assertive and passive, eager and afraid. In one kennel we saw two youngsters about four months old. The black Labrador pressed energetically against the cage door to greet us, but the other dog, a female Golden Labrador Retriever mix, waited shyly in the background.

We moved on to other cages and other dogs. We could not decide what to do. We walked past all the kennels again. Still we could not decide. We told Jennifer, the worker who had interviewed us, that we needed more time. She asked us to phone right away if we made a decision, since some dogs would not be there on Monday. We knew what she meant—they would be euthanized.

Then we left, weighed down by the plight of these homeless dogs and by our own inability to adopt one. We did not drive home, however, but went to Joyce's sculpture studio, which was nearby, and talked some more. That's when I said, "What about the puppy in the kennel with the black Lab?" We went back and asked to walk the Golden Lab. Jennifer brought her on a leash to give us some time with her alone. We took her outside for a stroll. When we stopped to pet her, Joyce crouched down and said, "Oh, you're such a sweet puppy." Reaching out an oversized paw, the puppy placed it on Joyce's knee, her vulnerable eyes singing "take my hand, lead me on, let me stand." We had been adopted.

We named our little dog after Rosa Luxemburg and Rosa Parks, two women who addressed the suffering of their generations. Later, when I visited the Civil Rights Museum in Memphis, I saw a bus like the one on which Rosa Parks refused to sit at the back. My self-guided tour ended at the motel room where The Reverend Martin Luther King Jr. had been shot and killed. As I read and reflected about the events leading to his assassination, I heard playing softly in the background Mahalia Jackson's recording of "Precious Lord, Take My Hand." Having a dog named Rosa helped us recall the courage and generosity of these pioneers for social justice.

Rosa Luxemburg Parks would also remind us of our adoption in the years ahead. Her favorite times at home, and mine too, were quiet weekends when I would read in the living room at 315 Benjamin Avenue, our cat Ebony on my lap, Rosa lying on the carpet nearby. Soon I would feel the soft nudge of Rosa's moist muzzle, and the adoption ceremony would begin again. First one big paw would drape over my knee to be stroked on its tender side. Rosa would gaze fondly like the Buddha, a picture of perfect contentment. A few minutes later, she would give me her other paw, and the silent song would continue.

In the first two months of Rosa's life with us I thoroughly revised the book manuscript for *Adorno's Aesthetic*

Theory. During long days at the computer in my on-campus office, Rosa was at my side. I finished the project in mid-July. To celebrate, Rosa and I went on a camping trip to P. J. Hoffmaster State Park, on the eastern shore of Lake Michigan—the first of many vacations the two of us would enjoy.

Rosa loved long hikes through the dunes and woods and along the shore of Lake Michigan. Every Sunday afternoon the two of us would drive to Hoffmaster or to one of the other wooded parks in West Michigan for a special outing. Lying patiently beside my desk, she would wait for the magic words: "Hey, Pups, shall we go for our big walk?" Then she would spring into action, eager for our next adventure.

One such adventure stands out from our first camping trip in mid-July 1990. As day turned into dusk, she and I sat along the beach to watch a glorious sunset over Lake Michigan. The brilliant sun slowly slid toward a liquid cradle, drawing shades of orange and indigo across the sky above. Inspired by magnificence, I was not ready for sleep. So Rosa and I hiked about three miles up the beach and three miles back. The woods between beach and campground had become pitch black by the time we returned. I had forgotten my flashlight and could not see a thing. "Rosa," I said to my seventh-month-old companion, "you need to find the path. I cannot see where to go." Rosa understood. Down the path she carefully padded, drawing me deftly along, leading me on to the light. We arrived at our campsite triumphant but tired.

Thirteen years later our roles reverse. Rosa has aged. Her vision is dim. Walking has become a challenge. We no longer hike at night. Even in full sunlight the day must seem to her "past and gone." In July 2004 we take our last camping trip together. It is not easy for Rosa. Weather disturbances make her anxious at night, and unexpected sounds unsettle her during the day.

Yet Rosa wants to hike the trails of Awenda Provincial Park on Ontario's Georgian Bay. As we walk I keep her on a short leash, not for her to guide me, but for me to steer her past unseen rocks and roots. Occasionally she stumbles. Yet she presses on. She is tired, she is weak, she is worn. Through the storm, through the night, I lead her on to the light: take her hand, precious dog, and lead her home.

3

Retrieval

DESERT LIVING makes water precious. I grew up on a small farm in the agricultural valley of north-central California. Had there not been an elaborate system for irrigation, the region would have been like a desert. Specially designed reservoirs in the valley collected mountain runoff. From the reservoirs water coursed through canals and ditches to thirsty farmland all around. Every ten days or so during the summer Sharkey, the local ditch tender, came around to say he was opening the sluices to our dairy. The water would tumble into our ditch and spread from there across the pasture and almond orchard. Controlling the flow of water and repairing broken levees made farm irrigation a big event.

In those days the water reached us through canals and open ditches; in later years it would travel through pipelines underground. Every day during the hot and dusty summers we farm kids would head down the road to the main ditch. There we would spend hours at a time, exploring, sunbathing, and playing in the water of life.

I said goodbye to this experience after my family moved into the town of Escalon when I was twelve. Now I would swim in the outdoor pool at the local high school.

But crowded, chlorinated water was no match for the fresh adventure of an irrigation ditch in the country.

Thirty years later the adventure returned, when Rosa became a true water dog. She was one year old. Joyce and I were living in Toronto for a half year with my best friend Ron Otten. Labrador Retrievers like Rosa are known for their prowess in the water, and she had already played in many lakes and streams. But Rosa had not learned to swim long distances in order to fetch on command.

One windy day in early spring, Ron, Rosa, and I took a ferry to the islands that lie across from Toronto's downtown harbor. Four-foot waves rolled in from Lake Ontario. As we walked along the shore, Ron found a large stick for Rosa to fetch. He threw it ahead on the beach. She scampered after it and proudly trotted back for another round. Then he threw it into the shallow water. Rosa walked in just far enough to grab it and bring it back. With each toss, Ron flung the stick a little farther. Rosa would walk as far as possible, swim a short distance to snatch the prize, and quickly return. Finally Ron thought "Let's go for it." He heaved the stick as far out as he could. Rosa could not see it, and I worried she might lose her way. But Ron urged her on.

Then it happened. Rosa plunged into the water, powering through the waves toward a goal she could not see. On and on she swam, until she found the object of her quest. She grabbed hold, turned around, and headed directly back to where we stood on the shore. With lavish praise Ron and I celebrated her baptism into the family of mature water dogs. Never again could we visit a lake without Rosa's insisting on repeated long-distance retrievals, no matter how high the waves or how cold the water.

Several years later Rosa baptized me. I did not need to learn how to swim, of course, and her joy at the beach often brought me into the water. Yet we had never swum together. One day her enthusiasm for fetching was too contagious. I could not resist. Throwing a stick, I plunged in with her and swam alongside, timing my strokes to make sure she arrived at our object first. Once she had seized the stick, we returned together. As we swam I could observe just how smooth and strong were her practiced strokes, as smooth and strong in water as I would like to be in life.

Eventually Rosa learned to go into the water without fetching, just for the pleasure of our swimming together. Passers by must have scratched their heads at the sight: a silly middle-aged man—a professor of philosophy, no less!—frolicking in Lake Michigan with his mature water dog. But I did not care. Rosa had helped me reclaim a childlike sense of adventure amid the pressures of academic work.

The day came when I could not let Rosa swim. By then she was a canine senior citizen. She had not lost the desire to swim, but the polluted lake water was too hard on her digestive system. During our last camping trip we did not swim at all. Instead we sat together on the Dog Beach at Awenda Provincial Park and watched the other dogs fetching. It pained me to be there and not let Rosa enjoy the water, for fear of the illnesses she so easily contracted. As she quietly gazed toward the horizon, I felt forlorn. Neither of us entered the water that day.

I returned to Awenda two years later, and more than a year after Rosa died. I camped across from the site of our last camping trip together. I sat by myself near the campfire at night and remembered our shared adventures. I revisited the trails where Rosa and I had hiked. Then I walked down to the Dog Beach alone. I sat there and thought about the happy times, saddened now by Rosa's death. I took out my diary and began to write. As memories, songs, and images came flooding in, the idea of a book began to take shape. It would be a book about Rosa, a book about loss and longing to be sure, but also about rebirth and new life. It would have as many chapters as she had years to live. It would be a personal testament to the baptism she gave me.

Suddenly the book's outline emerged, like a stick flung by a friend into the rocking waves. I closed my diary and put it away. I got up and looked at the distant horizon. Then I plunged into the water and swam. I swam, and I swam, and still I swim, into the water of life. With the memory of Rosa both waiting and watching, I venture farther than ever before. I return refreshed to the shore.[3]

4

Comfort

Dad was a peace-loving person and a man of few words. He bore the marks of someone who had suffered loss at an early age. Dad's mother died when he was five. Her death left my Grandpa Zuidervaart with six children from two mothers, three whose mother died when they were in school, and another three whose mother died when my father, the oldest, was not yet in school. A housekeeper and the older children helped my grandfather rear his family.

At age eleven, after only six years of schooling, my father left the parental home in a Dutch village outside Rotterdam to live and work on a nearby farm. To escape poverty and find new opportunities, he and his siblings then emigrated from the Netherlands. Dad was eighteen. He found work on a dairy farm in southern California and spent nearly two decades as a hired hand. When he had finally saved enough money to buy his own herd of cows, he married a woman from a large Dutch immigrant family of modest means. I was born four years later, the youngest of three children, and grew up on a small dairy in north-central California. Dad was in his early forties when I was born.

Although poor and not well schooled, both of my parents loved classical music. Every December they would sing Händel's *Messiah* with the Ripon Oratorio Society, my mother a sturdy alto and my father a lyric tenor. Although Dad was a chorus member in these performances, and not a soloist, I have always heard the opening tenor aria as his voice. It is the voice of someone acquainted with grief who does not complain: "'Comfort, comfort ye my people,' says your God."

This association comes, perhaps, from a forgotten experience in infancy. My mother used to tell the story, confirmed by others in my childhood church, about our family's attending a performance of *Messiah*. I was two. One would expect a toddler to become restless long before the end of a three-hour concert. But not little Lambert. Like his calm and patient father, he sat through the entire performance in rapt attention—not a peep out of him, my mother would say. I sat quietly for so long because I was on my father's lap. "Comfort, comfort ye my people."

I left this rural setting in California to attend university when I was eighteen, and I have never lived there since. Yet I have returned for frequent visits over the years. When Rosa was two years old Joyce and I rented a van to drive from Michigan to California and back. We wanted to introduce Rosa to my California family and friends. I was in my early forties at the time. Rosa rode reluctantly in the back of the van: she did not like being a passenger under the best of circumstances. Yet whenever we stopped she was eager for the next exploration.

On the return trip from visiting my California family, we three took the northern route, through Utah and Idaho to Grand Teton and Yellowstone National Parks. Although it was mid-June, the weather in Yellowstone was overcast and cold. Old Faithful shot out more steam than spray that day. As we headed to the west exit late in the afternoon, snow began to fall. The road turned slushy, then icy. It seemed to narrow with each darkening mile. Eventually we met a roadblock. Snow had closed the west exit. We would have to turn around.

By then Rosa, who always sensed our tension, had had enough. The sleeping bags wedged between the driver and passenger's seat posed no barrier. She pushed them aside and tried to crawl in front. Because I was driving, Joyce climbed into the back to hold and soothe her. But Rosa was too distraught, and Joyce could not restrain her. Soon our seventy-five-pound Golden Lab wormed her way under my feet. I had to stop the van. Then we decided to switch places. Joyce would drive; I would navigate from the passenger's seat; and Rosa, desperate Rosa, would sit on my lap.

It turned out that the only lodging available overnight was back in Grand Teton, a ninety-minute drive in hazardous conditions. With Joyce driving the treacherous route back, we sang to our panicky puppy. Hymns, folk songs, and lullabies we sang, as the minutes and miles crept by. And Rosa became calm, like a child on daddy's lap. She sighed, and pushed her head deep under my arm. Joyce and I felt less vulnerable too, less fragile, amid the giant boulders and jagged edges and slippery paths. The mutual consolation of a canine companion brought comfort to her people.

5

Fragile

On and on the rain will fall
Like tears from a star, like tears from a star
On and on the rain will say
How fragile we are, how fragile we are[4]

ROSA ENJOYED vigorous pursuits. No squirrel felt safe in our backyard. The deer in parks we visited had to run for their lives if she caught their scent. She brought the same enthusiasm to games with her human pack. When we lived in Toronto in 1991, Ron Otten and I went ice-skating in High Park on Grenadier Pond. We brought Rosa along. First she ran alongside us as we skimmed over the frozen water. Soon, however, and to the delight of other skaters, she was pulling me around the circle like a sled dog, with Ron racing ahead like a rabbit to chase.

Ron moved to the Netherlands a year later. In his absence, soccer balls became a special object of pursuit. Rosa regularly found them on our late-afternoon walks. Off leash in Wilcox Park in Grand Rapids, where school children often played, she would suddenly dash into the bushes. "Must be a squirrel," I thought. "Hope it has an emergency exit."

But, no, somehow Rosa had smelled an abandoned soccer ball. Back she trotted, tail waving proudly, the ball firmly gripped in her powerful jaws.

Soon Rosa's enthusiasm for soccer balls turned into a favorite sport. "Drop it," I would say. Then, "Back up! Back up!" As she pranced away, getting ever more excited, I would feint left, then right, then left again. She mirrored my movements like a professional goalie, anticipating the inevitable kick. As the ball sailed away, she lunged for the treasured prey, quickly pouncing on it or stopping it in mid-flight. Then she would bring me the soccer ball and prepare for round two.

But mad dashes did not always have happy endings. Late one afternoon when Rosa was nearly three years old, we went for a walk through the campus of Aquinas College, which borders Wilcox Park. As we hiked along a wooded stream, she scared up a rabbit and gave excited chase. Suddenly she stopped, as if yanked by an invisible leash, and limped back. Rosa could not put any weight on her left rear paw. I looked at it but could see nothing wrong—no cuts, no thorns, no obviously broken bones. "Must have sprained her leg," I thought. As we made our way home, Rosa sat every ten paces or so to lick her paw.

When we finally we arrived home, I called our animal clinic. They advised me to wait until morning to see whether Rosa's condition improved. I fixed supper and tried to make her comfortable. She could not settle in one spot for long. After an hour she started to whine and whimper, which she usually never did. So I examined her paw again. This time I saw something protruding ever so slightly between the third and fourth pads of the injured paw. It looked like a bone out of place. I could feel something rounded stretching for several inches under her skin. Was it a serious fracture? Had something jammed itself into her foot? She must be in considerable pain, I realized, and would need immediate attention.

By then the animal clinic had closed for the day, so I brought Rosa to an emergency clinic. The veterinarian there confirmed my worst fears. Rosa needed surgery under full anesthesia. Twenty minutes later she emerged from surgery sporting a bright green leg bandage and looking quite bewildered. Then the veterinarian showed me what she had found: a five-inch stick, in places nearly as thick as my little finger. Somehow during Rosa's mad dash the stick had jammed through her foot and into her leg until only the tip of the stick was showing.

I brought Rosa home and lifted her out of the car. Once inside the house, she lay down in the living room at our feet. Then from deep within her arose a piteous cry, part wail and part moan, over and over, until one's heart could break for this wounded creature. Joyce and I took turns lying beside her to give her the little comfort we could. We could do nothing to take away her trauma and pain.

What we could not offer was provided for us. Just three days later, Rosa tried to chase squirrels from our backyard, reminding them, in case they had forgotten, whose domain it really was. But what I remember most is not the quick recovery but her suffering, and the tears she could not shed. Many years later, after she died, they would be cried, on and on, like tears from a star—her unshed tears streaming from my face, saying, like the rain, how fragile we are.

In Toronto, on Rosa's last Sunday with us, she and I returned from our weekly "big walk" to a house full of people. It was February 2005. Women friends of Joyce and our goddaughter Esther Hart had gathered belatedly to celebrate Esther's thirty-seventh birthday one month earlier. Esther had been diagnosed with colon cancer during the previous year and had undergone extensive surgery and chemotherapy. We had celebrated the first birthday of Esther and David's daughter Sophie in December.

Rosa was very tired when she and I arrived home. After greeting the birthday party guests, I carried her upstairs to my second-floor study and prepared for a graduate seminar the next day. When everyone else had left, I heard a soft knock on the closed office door. I opened it. There was Esther. She wanted to tell me goodbye. Before leaving the room, she knelt down to talk to Rosa too. Maybe Esther sensed that Rosa did not have long to live, understood in her own illness how fragile we are. Esther never saw Rosa again.

Now it is ninth months later, in November 2005. Sophie's second birthday will be next week; soon midwinter snow will fall. Sophie and Esther and David are at our house for an American Thanksgiving dinner. Connie and Darlene have joined us from Grand Rapids, and Darlene's sister Wilhelmina has enjoyed dinner with us too. After supper we sit in the living room and talk. Sophie wants to play the piano in the adjoining room. So Joyce helps Sophie onto the piano bench and sits beside her.

As the two of them doodle at the keyboard, Sophie begins to fuss. She is tired and out of sorts. Joyce, who has been taking care of Sophie every weekday during Esther's illness, knows exactly what to do. She subtly slides into a beautiful piano rendition of "Twinkle, Twinkle, Little Star." As if by magic, the adults in the living room begin to hum the familiar tune. Soon we are singing in four-part harmony: "Twinkle, Twinkle, little star; how I wonder what you are." As Sophie listens from the piano bench, a puzzled peace dawns on her face. Our unplanned lullaby has soothed her spirit.

But Sophie does not know, as we adults do, that her mother Esther may not have long to live. If our absent Rosa could listen to our singing, perhaps she would hear the unshed tear. It twinkles in our eyes like a distant star, saying how fragile we are, how fragile we are.

6

Snow on Snow

> In the bleak midwinter, frosty wind made moan,
> earth stood hard as iron, water like a stone;
> snow had fallen, snow on snow, snow on snow,
> in the bleak midwinter, long ago.
>
> What can I give him, poor as I am?
> If I were a shepherd, I would bring a lamb;
> if I were a wise man, I would do my part;
> yet what I can I give him—give my heart.[5]

MIDWINTER SEEMED bleak until Rosa arrived. We seldom saw snow in California's agricultural flatlands where I grew up. From December to February, however, tule fog would rise ghostlike from warm soil and marshlands. It blanketed the valley for weeks at a time. Smudge pots lit to protect almond buds from killing frost would turn the fog into an impenetrable grey. Melancholy and depression were constant companions.

Yet not even this training in bleakness prepared me for the overcast cold of Grand Rapids, where one January we saw the sun only four hours in the entire month. Blowing lake-effect snow, dumped on us from neighboring Lake

Michigan, kept me indoors for days on end. Midwinter in Grand Rapids seemed desolate indeed.

Rosa changed all that. Like other dogs of her breed, she was an outdoor enthusiast and welcomed water in any form. Each winter she would celebrate the first snowfall by flinging herself down and rolling out a dog angel. No day was too cold for a romp in the snow, no sky too grey for a vigorous walk. Calling me daily into the damp outdoors, Rosa taught me to embrace the cold, to revel in the snow, to live into the bleakest midwinter.

Photographs from this time take me back to a Sunday afternoon in late February 1994. On previous days snow has fallen, snow on snow, snow on snow. But today the sky is crystalline and cloudless. I have my camera along. As Rosa and I hike across the dunes at P. J. Hoffmaster State Park, brilliant sunlight etches stark tree-shadows across the forest floor, latticing dusky grey on glistening white. We meander through the empty campgrounds where we have enjoyed many summer stays. Finally we clear the last hill. Below us spread the shoreline, the accumulated ice fields, and the frigid lake beyond. We hear no human sound, just the swish splash, swish splash, of rocking waves against jagged ice.

As Rosa and I walk to the beach, I see a hollow where a birch tree has smashed into the wooden railing along the hillside path. We clamber down. There we sit and rest. A branch just above us, its underside bare, drips melting snow, enshrined by the lapidary sky beyond. I photograph the branch from several angles. Then I turn toward Rosa. She stands like a sentinel in the snow, tiny ice droplets on her lower muzzle, the essence of patient eagerness. "I'll enjoy this eternal moment so long as you do," she seems to say.

"But when you come to your senses you will discover what a glorious romp awaits us on the ice fields below, where earth stands hard as iron, water like a stone."

Eleven years later, and many miles away, Rosa and I take another Sunday walk. Again we are in the bleak midwinter, this time at Sherwood Park in Toronto. One of the largest protected natural areas left in the heart of the city, Sherwood Park normally is a dog-walker's delight. White pine, hemlock, beech, oak, and sugar maples cover hillsides across which off-leash trails meander. But snow and freezing rain during the past week have coated the paths and trees with icy sheaths. Today the walking conditions are tricky for the able-bodied, and even more so for a large dog that has just turned fifteen and can no longer climb our household stairs.

The roadway down into the park is covered with salt. So we walk on the snow alongside the road and go up and down a few hills to avoid the salt. Rosa stumbles a few times but does not fall. The main trail for dog walking through the woods is very slippery. We proceed slowly, cautiously. Rosa slips twice on a very icy patch. A little farther I decide that the hills and steps are too treacherous. So we double back. We pause before the iciest patch to let other dogs and people pass us.

Then I figure out a way to avoid the ice by going off trail up the hill. I lift Rosa over a log along this detour. We slowly make our way to the end of the trail. There we come across a patch of soft snow. As if in celebration for having made it this far, Rosa flops down, rolls onto her back, and kicks like a little puppy. Two days later she would die.

By then Rosa had taught me what I would not have learned on my own. She did not let the cold enfold me. She showed me how to live into days when frosty wind made moan. What incredible strength and determination she shared, until the day she died. She continued daily routines without complaint, ever ready for a walk no matter how treacherous the conditions, always wanting to be near me in the house even when a spot to settle was hard to find.

Once, on a camping trip with Rosa, Ron and I talked late into the night about our hopes and sorrows. I told him then about my image of growing old: "I picture myself as a decrepit octogenarian, wheelchair-bound on a deserted hill, about whom no one gives a damn." Many years later, reflecting on Rosa's life and death, I have a different image. When I become an elderly companion to others, I want to be as gracious and generous as she. Decrepit and frail, no longer in my prime, may I not despair. May I remember instead Rosa's answer to bleak midwinter. What shall I give then? Give my heart.

7

Blessing

The trouble began when Rosa was five years old, a vigorous dog in her prime. Rosa loved our weekly long walks along the shore of Lake Michigan. This Sunday afternoon was crisp and cold. The snow-laden woods sparkled. We had hiked several miles through the dunes and along the beach, basking in the serene sunlight. Now it was time to return through the dunes and drive back home.

We had barely left the beach when Rosa collapsed without a sound. Her hind legs gave out; she sank onto her haunches in the snow. Thinking she had slipped into a hidden hole, I urged her to get up. She made no effort in response. I tugged gently on her leash. She gave me a quizzical look, but did not budge. Then I knew something was wrong, but had no explanation. What should I do? Could I carry our seventy-five-pound beauty for more than a mile on a hilly, snow-covered trail? We waited and wondered. After several minutes, Rosa struggled to her feet, and we resumed our homeward trek.

Rosa would show ever-stronger signs of discomfort in the months ahead. She developed a limp. It became harder for her to get up and lie down. Her play became less vigorous, although she remained eager for the outdoors. I feared our Sunday walks would never be the same.

Several months later, not long after Easter, Fountain Street Church invited people in Grand Rapids to celebrate Reverence for Life Sunday. The morning service would include the church's annual Blessing of the Animals. People would bring all manner of pets into the sanctuary to be blessed—cats and dogs, to be sure, but also birds, snakes, and llamas. This was a big event in the community, but Joyce and I had never attended. We decided to take part, with Rosa at our side. One after another people and their companion animals filed to the front of the church where two pastors greeted them. Rosa and I joined the procession.

Going forward in a liturgical procession, no matter how irregular and informal, was foreign to my experience. I grew up in a religious tradition that prized sobriety. There were only two sacraments—baptism and communion—and these were observed, not celebrated. Evangelical altar calls never occurred either. I remember my embarrassment at my father's enthusiasm every Easter Sunday when the congregation of my childhood church would sing "Low in the Grave He Lay," a nineteenth-century hymn by Robert Wadsworth Lowry. The song begins with a plaintive meditation. At the chorus, however, it jumps into a jubilant march: "Up from the grave He arose, with a mighty triumph o'er His foes." My dad, who had lost his Dutch mother when he was five and whose closest brother died not long after they immigrated to California, always leapt into this chorus, leading the congregation by an entire beat. You could hear his clear and passionate "Up" before everyone else, a sly subversion of Calvinist sobriety by a gentle man for whom death could not have the final word.

Perhaps this repeated experience at Easter shadowed me in the Fountain Street procession. Self-consciously, but with desperate hope, I went forward with Rosa. We came to the front of the line. A pastor asked, "What is your dog's name?" "Rosa, Rosa Luxemburg Parks." "And what is her ailment?" "She has arthritis in her back hips," I said. Placing his hands on her hindquarters, the pastor said, "Rosa, I bless your hips." That was it: the blessing of our animal. We walked back to the pew where Joyce waited, Rosa sniffing other pets along the way.

But that was not it, really. Affirmed by this blessing, we consulted with veterinarians; we had X-rays taken; we even considered surgery and canine acupuncture. In the end we found a human mineral supplement, sold over the counter, that helped regenerate the cartilage in Rosa's creaking joints. She would live for another ten years, frisking and frolicking through many of them, until she slowly succumbed to the aging of her muscles and bones.

Our many friends in Grand Rapids knew of Rosa's condition and of her miraculous recovery. After we had moved to Toronto, they continued to share our fondness for her lovely spirit. When Rosa died, Simona Goi, who had lost her own dog to a sudden illness a few years earlier, wrote us the following note of condolence:

> I am so very sorry to hear of Rosa's passing. She was truly a fantastic dog. All of us who knew her loved her. We all also know that she had the best possible life a dog could have. She never lacked for attention and affection; she got to do all

the things that dogs most enjoy: being around people, going for walks, having little jobs like carrying the paper, and occasionally snapping at those pesky cats!

I know it is really hard to lose such a lovely and trusted friend, but you should rest assured that no one could have taken better care of her, and that she lived a full and happy life. You were generous in being attentive to her wishes of being let go . . .

Right now she is probably very much thinking of you as she plays around in doggy heaven, where some defunct philosopher is always ready to let her carry his newspaper, while a very talented artist can't wait to have Rosa sit around in her studio while she sculpts. The only advantage in doggy heaven over doggy earth is that in heaven Rosa's hips are fabulous, and occasionally she even considers jumping for a Frisbee. I'm sure she'll show you that when you get to see her again . . .

See her again I shall, perhaps even on this doggy earth. Like my father on an Easter morning, Rosa will leap ahead, leading all our companions in a procession that never ends, a joyous blessing of the animals. Rosa will not stumble. And I shall be eager to follow, sobered by affliction and death, yet celebrating the renewal of life.

8

Rest Gently, Gently Rest

Wir setzen uns mit Tränen nieder
Und rufen dir im Grabe zu:
Ruhe sanfte, sanfte ruh'!
Ruht, ihr ausgesognen Glieder!
Ruhe sanfte, sanfte ruh'!
Euer Grab und Leichenstein
Soll dem ängstlichen Gewissen
Ein bequemes Ruhekissen
Und der Seelen Ruhstatt sein.
Höchst vergnügt schlummern da die Augen ein.

We sit down in tears
And call to you in the grave:
Rest gently, gently rest!
Rest, you worn-out limbs!
Rest gently, gently rest!
Your grave and headstone
Will offer the troubled soul
A pleasant pillow
And the heart a place of rest.
With utter joy our eyes close in sleep.

I

The chorus that ends Bach's *St. Matthew Passion* brings comfort amid sadness.[6] The Crucified One rests in a sealed-up tomb, rocked by a double choir of angels, as an orchestral universe keeps solemn watch. No one who has lost a loved one will escape the grief mixed with compassion, like blood and water from a wounded side, that here flow mingled down.

Listening to this music brings me back to February 1989, the day after my father's funeral. I go to the cemetery alone, afternoon already slipping toward dusk. Burwood District Cemetery is a familiar spot. The farm where I grew up lies just across the road. Often we neighborhood kids would help Mr. Allen, the cemetery caretaker, remove faded flowers from gravesites. When Mr. Allen was on vacation in my teenage years, I would replace him, maintaining the grounds, selling plots, and digging and filling graves. It is a lovely place. Stately oak trees and elms shade the lawn and shrubs, creating a green oasis amid farm-country dust.

Today I am inconsolable. The father I had always hoped to know better has died after a massive stroke left him mute and helpless. I struggled during his three-month hospitalization to find ways to express my love. I did not know what he could understand. Now, standing at his grave, I say aloud what it seems only I can hear. "Goodbye, Dad," I whisper. "We'll see each other in a better life where you won't suffer, and you won't be oppressed, and we'll share everything we want to share. Goodbye." —We sit down in tears / And call to you in the grave: / Rest gently, gently rest!

I walk back to the car and get in. As I sit collecting myself, a golden-haired dog appears. It walks over the hillside from the direction of our former farm. I have never seen the dog before. It trots directly to the car and stops on the passenger side, just far enough away to look me in the eye. I feel myself in the presence of a great mystery. I get out of the car and begin to talk. The dog cocks its head and listens. Then it moves nearer, close enough for me to reach out and scratch its head. I tell the dog about Dad: "Just over there lies a man who loves animals. He would not mind if you lie down beside his grave." —Rest, you worn-out limbs! / Rest gently, gently rest!

I return to the car. The dog follows for a few paces. When I close the door, it backs away from the car, far enough to see me again. I look at it. It looks at me. Then it walks in front of the car. Our eyes meet once more. The dog turns away. Without a backward glance it saunters up the hill and disappears, headed toward what had been my father's farm. Now hidden warmth spreads from deep inside. I know a peace that passes understanding. In wordless dialogue with a dog, at last I have heard my father's muted voice. And he has heard mine. —Your grave and headstone / Will offer the troubled soul / A pleasant pillow / And the heart a place of rest.

II

Joyce and I adopted our golden-haired Rosa one year later. I do not recall looking for a dog of a certain breed or size or color. You could say Rosa Luxemburg Parks found us just as much as we found her. But from the day we brought her home in May 1990, my dialogue with a dog continued. Often my words were spoken, to be sure, and on some occasions our dog was so verbal that we would call her Rosa Barks. The deeper connections, however, lay in unscripted moments of silent sharing. At night she always slept alongside our bed. —With utter joy our eyes close in sleep.

One February morning fifteen years later Rosa did not try to get up from her blanket when we awoke. She had been sleeping on the floor beside me. Her nest was a blanket we had bought during the late 1970s when I was doing my doctoral research in Berlin. Stitched into the Berlin blanket was the word "love." To turn the blanket into a wall hanging for our sparsely furnished student apartment, Joyce had woven woolen fringes across the word "love." Like my faltering efforts at Dad's bedside before he died, "love" was there, but hidden.

After inviting Rosa to come downstairs for breakfast, I went alone and started the coffee maker. When I came back to the bedroom, Rosa had not stirred. She was still in a flat-down position, front legs splayed to each side of her head, and back legs curled awkwardly beneath her. I decided to help her up and lifted her hindquarters. Her back legs dangled limply in mid air, and she did not use her front legs for leverage. She appeared to have suffered a stroke. Lowering her, I knew this might be the end.

Joyce was filling the bathtub for her bath. I walked into the bathroom and touched her shoulder: "Something is wrong with Rosa. She can't get up." We went to the bedroom together. I tried once more to help Rosa up, without success. "I think it's time," I said. "I think she's telling us she's ready to leave us." "Why don't you lie next to her and talk with her while I take my bath," Joyce replied. "Then let's call the vet's office to arrange a time when he can see her."

So I lay down next to Rosa and stroked her worn-out limbs. Her spine felt very tight, and her front legs passive. She kept her eyes half closed most of the time. She seemed to have lost her spirit. I softly sang a ditty I had made up in 1991 to sing to her when we rested during our daily walks.

> Rosa is a very fine dog,
> Yes, we love our Rosa.
> Rosa is a very fine dog,
> Yes, she is.

Then Joyce talked with Rosa as I took my bath. Around 7:30 I left a message on the answering machine at the Woodbine Animal Clinic.

Shortly after 9:00 Joyce called the vet again. The receptionist said we could bring Rosa in right away. I got the car ready and opened the back door of the house. Then I went back upstairs, where Joyce was sitting with Rosa. "This is our last goodbye, Pups," I said. "We're going to see the doctor," Joyce told her. "You like the doctor."

Tenderly we lifted Rosa in the Berlin love nest on which she lay. Rosa accepted this without struggle. We carried our precious Pups downstairs, out the door, and into the back seat of the car for one last ride. I sat with her and stroked her as Joyce drove us to the clinic. Once there we carried Rosa directly into the examining room and laid her, blanket and all, on the metal table. Dr. Littlejohn came into the room and talked with us. He confirmed our judgment that it was time to say goodbye. Rosa looked up a few times but barely raised her head.

Dr. Littlejohn called in his assistant and trimmed some fur off Rosa's front right leg. As my tears flowed, Joyce repeated softly "You're a good dog, Rosa. We love you, Pups. Thank you for being such a great dog." Silently I held Rosa's collar with one hand and caressed her head and neck with the other. Finally I could say, "You're a good dog, Rosa. We love you. Goodbye." The needle went in, the serum flowed into her, and a minute later Rosa was gone.

We did not linger. But Joyce had the great presence of mind to leave our blanket with Rosa. That is my lasting image of our sweet dog, resting gently, gently resting, wrapped in our blanket of love. Around her swells an angel chorus: Dad's voice, Rosa's voice, the voices of all loved ones lost and found. –We sit down in tears / And call to you in the grave: / Rest gently, gently rest! / Rest, you worn-out limbs! / Rest gently, gently rest!

9

Benediction

> Lascia ch'io pianga
> mia cruda sorte,
> e che sospiri la libertà.
> Il duolo infranga queste ritorte
> de' mei martiri sol per pietà.
>
> Leave me to weep
> over my cruel fate
> and let me sigh for liberty.
> May sorrow break the bonds of my anguish,
> if only for pity's sake.[7]

It is 4:00 a.m. the day after Rosa died. I am wide-awake from a brief and troubled sleep. Before going to bed last night I talked on the phone with my sister-in-law Brenda. She had called to let us know that my ninety-year-old mother, who lives alone in our family's home, is suffering from pain in her leg and hip. Until last month Mom was riding her bicycle around Escalon twice a day. But then she fell off her bike and collapsed twice in her own house. Now for the first time Mom is walking with a cane. She will need to enter an assisted care facility. We will have to sell the family home.

Shortly before Brenda called, as I looked at pictures of Rosa in our photo albums, CBC radio broadcast a song that sent tears streaming down my face. Soprano Hélène Guilmette, accompanied by the Montreal-based Les Violons du Roy, sang "Lascia ch'io pianga," a hauntingly lovely aria from Händel's Italian opera *Rinaldo*: "Leave me to weep over my cruel fate and let me sigh for liberty. May sorrow break the bonds of my anguish, if only for pity's sake."

Rosa's death yesterday and Mom's aging weave through the three-part dream from which I have just awakened.

> Scene 1: I am at an outdoor family gathering. My brother Martin and I are playing tennis. The game is not going well. I am frustrated and embarrassed at my clumsy efforts. When I miss an easy return, we send Rosa off to fetch the tennis ball. She cannot find it. I go over to join the search and find the missing object for her. But she does not want to carry it back. So I toss it ahead for her to chase. Rosa takes only a couple of steps, then collapses in pain.
>
> Scene 2: My adult siblings and I are indoors now, but not at home. We have gathered for a family dinner. Mom asks whether one of us will offer a blessing before the meal. My sister Roelyn and I assume that Martin, the oldest sibling, will say a prayer. But he does not want to do it. As we awkwardly wait, Mom breaks into a powerful and beautiful song in Dutch. The others seem embarrassed, but I am deeply moved. I ask Mom about her song. She says it is the Dutch setting for Psalm 6. "When I was growing up," she explains, "my family often sang their prayers." The

> tune she sang is not a Dutch psalm setting, however. It is the melody to "Lascia ch'io pianga." In my dream Mom has offered a Kaddish for Rosa's departure.
>
> Scene 3: It is time for my family to go home. We agree that I will leave first and take the dogs with me in the car. But everyone is confused about when the others will head home and whether Mom will ride with the dogs and me. "That's no problem," I assure them. "I do not mind waiting at home for everyone else to arrive. I can always read."

I cannot ignore the irony in the third scene. As someone who took to academic and creative explorations early on, I have lived much of my life in intellectual pursuits. They have been my way to discover a much larger world than the rural community in which I grew up. Reading and writing have been my way to venture out. So even when my family arrives at the end of the dream, I will be taking my leave: "I can always read."

Yet this dream sequence also tells me that love for others sustains my explorations. I look for the tennis ball when Rosa cannot find it, and I toss it ahead in hope for her return. I welcome Mom's song, strange and old-fashioned though it be, and I receive it as a benediction. And, although I leave the gathering first, I do not go alone. Canine companions are with me. Nor do I break the family ties, but wait in my own fashion for everyone else to arrive. But why do I leave first? Perhaps from a desire to take care of loved ones beyond their own demise. Perhaps I want to create a place of love for them, a place where pain and suffering are no more, where God wipes the tears from every eye.

Psalm 6, sung by Mom in my dream, is a "penitential psalm." So far as I can remember, I have not heard or read it in years. The psalm pleads for mercy and healing. It asks God for deliverance because of God's "unfailing love." What dead person remembers God, the psalmist dares to ask. "Who praises you from the grave [*Sheol*]?" Next occurs a lament that one could set to Händel's tune:

> I am weary with my moaning;
> every night I flood my bed with tears;
> I drench my couch with my weeping.
> (Psalm 6:6, NRSV)

But where Händel's aria devolves into self-pity, the psalmist then breaks into jubilation: God has heard my cry, and my enemies will be disgraced:

> The LORD has heard my supplication;
> The LORD accepts my prayer.
> All my enemies shall be ashamed
> and struck with terror;
> They shall turn back,
> and in a moment be put to shame.
> (Psalm 6:9–10, NRSV)

Neither a song of self-pity nor a march of victory rings true after Rosa's death. I mourn for her, not only for myself, and no divine intervention will undo her collapse. Give me instead my mother's song. It turns both Händel's aria and Psalm 6 into a benediction.

Reflecting on the accidental death of his seventeen-year-old grandson Patrick, Bruce McLeod writes: "Love . . . is the permanent presence in God's world that refuses to give suffering the last word—with us in the worst of times, like a mother, hurt in our hurt, weeping with our tears, holding our rage and our pain and our asking Why. Never letting go, surprising our thin strength over and again with resilience we never guessed ahead of time was there."[8]

Love is the thread that stitches together my dreams. It is the refusal amid suffering to let go: to let go of life, to let go of hope, to let go of the ones I love most. Embraced by this refusal, I am free to take my leave. Rosa will go with me. I can always read.

10

Field of Love

> You'll remember me when the west wind moves
> Upon the fields of barley
> You can tell the sun in his jealous sky
> When we walked in fields of gold[9]

Early in December 2004 I e-mailed Ron Otten in Amsterdam. It was Ron who initiated Rosa into mature water doghood. "I am beginning to prepare myself for Rosa's departure," I wrote. "She'll be 15 in February . . . Her eyesight and hearing are not so sharp anymore. Lately she's been waking me up frequently at night for no apparent reason . . . This might be due to early stages of dementia, or simply Rosa's response to not being able to track her environment by sight and hearing. But she's still a sweet and beautiful dog. Putting her down, if that's what it comes to, will be one of the hardest decisions we'll ever make, and one of the hardest to live with later."

One month later Ron replied: "As I was walking in the woods last week, I suddenly felt the impending loss of Rosa. I remembered some of her gestures which always touched me, for example, the way she would so insistently and repeatedly place her big paw on my knee as a way of 'asking' me to do some of that 'deep-scratching' on the underside of her leg. And then that benign dog-like gazing into the distance off [to] the right or left as she enjoyed it.... If I can feel that it will be a loss when she dies, I can only imagine how hard it must be for you to part with her."

What Ron wrote next has stayed with me: "I have so much comfort in the Tibetan approach to death because it has helped me ... see that when a loved one dies, and Rosa is a loved one, that it's possible to do more than stand helplessly by, that it's possible to help her by creating a 'field of love' around her which supports her as her spirit 'moves on.'.... The love you and Rosa felt for each other survives death, and that is ... a genuine and powerful truth [and] a counterforce to so much tragedy in the world. The harmony and warmth which she helped bring into your lives were thereby also brought into the world at large, through you, through your work, through the letters you write to me, through the way in which guests are always welcomed into your home ... I hope that you can feel this undercurrent of the gift of her life and ... of her death ... that the painful loss of her dear and gentle companionship will be softened a little."

Seven weeks after I received Ron's e-mail, and one week after we celebrated her fifteenth birthday, Rosa died. When she died, I took Ron's wisdom to heart. Joyce and I created a "field of love" to surround Rosa's departure. I stopped working for several days. I revisited the paths I had most recently hiked with her. I listened to music that moves the spirit. I lit candles in Rosa's memory. I reviewed letters and photographs from the Rosa years and wrote in my journal. I corresponded with her many human friends. I cried, sometimes in Joyce's embrace, sometimes alone.

And, perhaps the most difficult step, in January 2006, eleven months after Rosa died, I joined a choir, for the first time in thirty years. Often the beauty of our harmony exposed such an ache in my heart that I could not sing. Yet I continued, not simply for my own sake or for the choir, but to help create Rosa's field of love.

A few days after Rosa's death Joyce and I received a framed photograph from our goddaughter Esther Hart. It hangs in my office at home. A gifted graphic designer, Esther had digitally altered a photograph taken by Henk Hart, her father and my predecessor at the graduate school where I teach philosophy. The photograph carries a penumbra of peace, due in part to its being slightly out of focus.

Henk took this picture on Canadian thanksgiving in 2003, which Joyce and Rosa and I spent with the Hart family. After dinner several of us went to a friend's farm to walk in the pumpkin fields and nearby woods. It was a gorgeous afternoon, seasoned in sunlight and spiced with care. An avid photographer, Henk had his digital camera along. The photograph he and Esther created shows Joyce and me walking in a field with Rosa. Joyce and I have our heads down in confidential conversation. Our backs are to the camera as we head toward autumnal trees cloaked in sunset colors. We have just stepped out of a large shadow and into the light. As Henk later wrote in an e-mail, our stepping into the light of evening surrounds us with an aura of calm. It speaks of peace as we face endings. It also speaks of readiness for new life.

In this photograph, where we face endings as new beginnings, Rosa walks beside me. She is tethered to a white rope. Her head up, she pulls away. But the sunlight glinting on a tether of white creates an ethereal effect: as she moves away, she remains firmly connected to us, as she always will be, ever with us in Rosa's field of love. We'll remember her when the west wind moves upon the fields of barley. And we'll tell the sun in a jealous sky when she walked in fields of gold.

11

Healing

WHEN JOYCE and I adopted Rosa in 1990, she was four months old, and I was nearly forty. My father had died in the previous year. He suffered a sudden stroke and never spoke again. Dad had been in excellent health, and I lived thousands of miles away. So I was not prepared for his demise. Because he was such a quiet man for whom English was a second language, I had never found the right time and place to verbalize my deepest affection. In the three months between the stroke and his death, I flew from Michigan to California several times. Dad could show only by an occasional gesture or smile that he might have understood what I was saying. He died one month after his eightieth birthday, the last time I saw him alive. I felt anguish because we never said a proper goodbye.

Rosa quickly showed herself an angel of mercy. Her playfulness and loyalty and affection brought healing to my troubled spirit. During the first years of her life Joyce and I attended Sunday morning worship with the Dominican Sisters at Marywood Chapel in Grand Rapids. We met in a modest light-filled room whose intimacy inspired quiet reflection. So did a folk hymn we often sang:

> Healer of our every ill,
> light of each tomorrow,
> give us peace beyond our fear,
> and hope beyond our sorrow.[10]

Sometimes I could only listen and hum along, tears in my eyes, a feeling of loss over Dad's death drowning the promise of restoration, a longing for peace deepening the sense of sorrow. But I could not give up hope for recovery, and Rosa's companionship helped relieve my sadness. I took to carrying a copy of the song's lyrics in my wallet during my long walks with her on Sunday afternoons. Our favorite spot was a secluded knoll where the somber rustling of stunted oak trees echoed the calm of Marywood Chapel. Seated high among the dunes overlooking Lake Michigan, with Rosa lying nearby, I would whisper to her the plaintive tune: "Healer of our every ill, light of each tomorrow . . ." Then we would quietly gaze across the wooded dunes and vast lake toward an indistinct line where sky meets water.

When Rosa died many years later, Joyce and I asked to have her cremated. I recall vividly the day one week later when we picked up her ashes. As the midwinter sun fades, Joyce and I walk to Woodbine Animal Clinic to claim Rosa's remains. Upon our return home we pour ourselves scotch and light candles in the living room. Then I unpack the urn containing the ashes of our beautiful dog. The urn has a sandy texture. It is brownish-grey with gold flecks, the colors of the beach and dune grasses in autumn, when Rosa and I used to take a special mid-semester camping trip and we would sit on our secluded knoll.

I propose a toast to Rosa, our beautiful, gentle, wise, and loving companion. Then Joyce gives me a framed print by Doug Guildford titled "A Boy and His Dog." The earth-tone print has five russet images, partially abstracted like paper cutouts, against a beige backdrop. In one the dog and boy play fetch; in another the dog sits on the boy's lap; in a third image boy and dog lie down to wrestle; in the next the dog kicks up its back legs as the boy tosses a ball between upraised hands; and in the fifth panel the dog crouches and barks as the boy high-steps over it. Tears well up when I unwrap Joyce's gift. I can barely speak, except to say, "It's lovely." Through her own tears, while hugging me, Joyce tells me how much it has meant to her to see me become playful again, thanks to Rosa. And Joyce is right. Rosa's companionship helped save my life. Rosa did not let me continue to wallow in anguish over my father's death. Playing with her and training her and receiving her affection gave me hope beyond my sorrow.

Two months later, during a weekend visit in Grand Rapids, I hike into Hoffmaster State Park with our friend Daryl. After Daryl turns back to take her dog Gibson to his veterinary appointment, I continue to the quiet knoll atop a dune where Rosa and I often contemplated the world. An oak tree, its trunk buried in the shifting sand, extends its main branches in five directions. A nest of dune grasses fills the hollow where the branches meet the buried trunk. I dig out a piece of sod. I gently place a remembrance of Rosa in the hollow. It is a special matchbox Ron had given me years ago. Inside the matchbox is Rosa's dog tag from 2001, our last complete year in Michigan before we moved to Toronto. I have wrapped it in a note of gratitude for the fifteen wonderful years we shared.

The only other witness is a small ceramic figurine, given to me the day before by our good friend Connie. Her sister Lucie made it based on photographs of Rosa. I call the figurine "Little Rosa." Little Rosa looks on as I say goodbye. She cannot speak, no more than my father could after his stroke, and no more than can the cremated ashes of our precious pet. But that does not matter.

Wind from the west stirs the browning oak leaves, remnants of seasons past. Before putting the sod back in place, I sing into the wind. I sing a song of Benjamin. I sing of light and peace and hope. They come to me now, shimmering off Lake Michigan, dog-kissing me through the tears. And Little Rosa knows, as her namesake knew, what the singer now also knows: no affliction can separate us, neither stroke nor death, from a wordless love that heals every ill.

12

Reunion

Growing up on a small dairy, I was surrounded by animals: cows and calves, chickens and ducks, cats and dogs. We children understood the difference between farm animals and pets, and we learned to respect and care for them all. The cows needed to be herded, milked, and fed. Occasionally a cow would let us ride on its back when my dad wasn't looking, but we knew it was not a pet: its purpose was to bear calves and give milk. The calves could be endearing, even when they bucked their pails of milk at feeding time, but they were groomed for milking or sold. The chickens and ducks never became our pets either, although we children took care of them and collected their eggs. Eventually the chickens themselves would end up on the kitchen table. For the most part the cats lived outside, hunted mice, and lapped up fresh milk when my dad fed them in the barn. Rarely did they become household pets. Only the dogs were companion animals, although they too spent most of their time outdoors.

This boundary blurred, however, when my parents bought three little goats. The goats were adorable speckled creatures, nimble of foot and full of mischief. I do not know whether they were part of a new business venture, but my siblings and I claimed one each as a pet. I was very fond of all three. Their intelligence and energy made them wonderful companions for a six-year-old boy who was the youngest child. Intelligence and energy also made the goats hard to keep fenced in. Repeatedly they found paths to freedom and romped through my mother's flowers. Eventually she had enough of their mischief and declared they would have to go. My father, who did not like conflict, agreed to bring them to market.

Our farmhouse sat on a sandy hill that sloped through an almond orchard to an open field below. It was a Saturday, as I recall, when the fateful hour neared. Perhaps to hide the goats, or perhaps to say farewell in my own place and on my own terms, I released all three from their frequently rebuilt pen and led them down the hill. There I sat, petting them, talking with them, and awaiting an inevitable departure. Their departure was unbearably harsh. Because we were too poor to own a pickup truck, our family car would have to do. Their nimble feet bound, the goats were put into the trunk of the car. They bleated helplessly as my dad drove away. I had no way to save them. It was like losing a family. I have felt their loss ever since.

Five decades later the little boy in me still dreaded the unavoidable departure of an animal companion. Rosa had lived with Joyce and me for fifteen years—as I said in the preface to my book *Artistic Truth*, a constant source of sanity and delight. I knew that when Rosa died the months ahead would be long and hard. For them to be a time of farewell, and not simply of loss, I could no longer look on helplessly as a companion left me behind.

When I was twelve my parents sold the farm and our family moved into Escalon, a small town about three miles away. We settled into a spacious ranch-style home on a tree-lined street called Sierra Drive. There I lived my teenaged years, and there I returned from distant places for family visits after I left home at the age of eighteen. The house on Sierra Drive became the new center of my family's universe.

Three months after Rosa died I traveled to California to begin preparations to sell the family home. Mom had moved into an assisted care facility one month earlier. She was able to return home for the duration of my final stay. Both a faithful letter writer and a proverbial pack rat, Mom had accumulated countless boxes and drawers of cards and letters, including all of my monthly letters since 1968. We reminisced, and she answered questions as I sorted through her lifelong correspondence. It was a special time.

On the Sunday morning of my visit I accompanied Mom to my childhood church. After lunch, as she read and rested in the living room, I decided to play a medley of psalms and hymns for her, as I had often done as a teenaged pianist. The old spray-painted piano, purchased used when my sister and I began lessons five decades earlier, was badly out of tune. Nevertheless, I threw myself into the music and hoped it would bring Mom joy.

The piano stood in the family room on one end of the house, separated by a kitchen and a dining room from the living room where Mom sat. The doors between these rooms were open, and I assumed that Mom was listening. To end the recital I gave a heartfelt rendition to one of her favorite hymns. Its fourth verse reads: "When we are called to part, it gives us inward pain; but we shall still be joined in heart, and hope to meet again."[11]

As I ended my medley, Mom walked into the family room. "Oh, there you are," she said. "I thought you were taking a nap." Her hearing was so impaired that she had not heard a single note! I had really been playing songs for myself, and perhaps for a community of kindred spirits.

These experiences have come together in a dream I recorded a few months after Rosa died. I am driving a car along a country road. My parents and brother and sister are passengers. Rosa is in the car too. Now the road winds onto a cliff that becomes ever more narrow as we go. The cliff drops away sharply on either side. One mistake and the car will plunge to destruction.

Eventually we come to a large hole in the road. I stop the car, get out, and look. We cannot to go forward. Nor can I turn the car around. There is barely enough room for everyone else to get out. But cautiously, painstakingly, they do. I discover a steep path wending down one side of the cliff to a farmhouse far below. My family slowly descends.

Rosa, however, is too old and frail to make the journey. I do not hesitate. I know what to do. Lovingly I lift her. Trusting me, Rosa makes not a sound. I carry her downward, downward, never stopping, never stumbling, until she and I reach the open field below. Then, to my surprise, I do not put her down. I clutch her to my chest, like a goatherd carrying a lost kid home, and walk onward to a glad farmhouse reunion. There the dream ends. Yet I know who awaits us inside. It is the family I lost as a child.

13

Alone

> Did you ever see a robin weep
> When leaves begin to die?
> That means he's lost his will to live
> I'm so lonesome I could cry
>
> The silence of a falling star
> Lights up a purple sky
> And as I wonder where you are
> I'm so lonesome I could cry[12]

Rosa did not enjoy car rides. Yet traveling was part of her routine: weekly outings to distant parks, frequent camping trips during the summer and fall, and extended vacations with friends and relatives in far-flung places. She also grew used to our moving. She was less than a year old when we moved to Toronto for a half year and then back to West Michigan. When she was three, we moved five blocks from 515 Norwood Avenue to 315 Benjamin in Grand Rapids. Nine years later we relocated permanently to Toronto. And before that we had spent a summer in Boston and a sabbatical year in Toronto. At each place Rosa quickly settled into her new environment. But she found certain disruptions hard: when we left her behind during our travels, and when everything disappeared into a moving van. I have two vivid memories of this.

In May 1996 I traveled to Europe for twelve days to attend a conference in Prague and to visit Ron Otten in Amsterdam. From Amsterdam I flew to Toronto for several days of meetings and visits with friends. Joyce met me there, having left Rosa with Donna and Bill in Grand Rapids. Joyce and I drove back to Grand Rapids on June 2. By then Rosa had not seen me for more than two weeks.

Rosa enjoyed staying with Donna and Bill. They lavished on her all the affection a lovable dog could want. Yet she missed her pack, and we missed her. Driving into Grand Rapids, Joyce and I were so eager to see Rosa that we went directly to Donna and Bill's house before going home. No one answered our soft knocking, however, and Rosa must have been sound asleep. We peeked through a window. There lay our peaceful Pups lolling in the sunlight on the dining room floor. She was completely oblivious to our return. Rather than disturb her beauty rest, we quietly went home and waited there for Donna and Bill to phone.

Two hours later we received the welcome call and hurried back. Donna answered the door, with Rosa right behind her, tail wagging but eyes subdued. As I stepped inside, Rosa nestled her head against my legs and held it there for the longest time. Then, with affectionate licks to the hand, she reclaimed me. "You may disappear from time to time," she seemed to say, "but I will never let you go."

My other memory comes from our permanent move to Toronto in June 2002. It was a large undertaking. We had to pack up everything, including Joyce's sculpture studio and my on-campus office, for transportation and customs-clearance to another country. It meant leaving behind a large and lovely house in a neighborhood where we felt fully at home.

As each room emptied, Rosa became more downcast. The last room to empty was our living room, where Rosa had welcomed so many guests and students over the years, and where she often rested near my favorite chair. Late that afternoon when the movers drove away, there Rosa lay, the only occupant left in the largest and once the liveliest room of the house, looking so lonesome she could cry.

To cheer her up, I asked whether she wanted to go for a walk—an occurrence before suppertime that she usually welcomed. Today, however, she would not budge. Only when Joyce agreed to walk with us would Rosa leave the house. The same thing happened when we stayed at our friends' house that night. At bedtime I asked Rosa whether she wanted to go out for a walk. She went to the door eagerly, but would not leave the front steps. Once Joyce joined us, however, Rosa gladly sauntered down the sidewalk. The same pattern continued for the first few days in Toronto before our furniture arrived. To have all the familiar things of her household disappear during the course of one long day had been too much. Rosa was afraid of losing one of us too.

The summer after Rosa died in 2005 I had no desire to go camping. I would rather stay in our strangely silent house than enjoy the outdoors without her. Like Rosa on the day of our big move, I did not want to leave my companion behind. For the first time since she had joined our household, I stayed home all summer. It felt as if I had lost the will to live.

Not until early October, at the end of the camping season, was I ready to venture out alone. It was the weekend before Canadian Thanksgiving. The weather was cold and grey at Ontario's Pinery Provincial Park on the eastern shore of Lake Huron. Very few people were around. After setting up camp in the chilling damp, I went for a hike on the Carolinian Trail. It winds up and down the dunes in one of the few remaining stands of Carolinian forest. My previous time there, in May 2004, Rosa had been along. Now, walking the trail alone, I could picture the two of us laboring up the dune stairways, stopping to rest as I read about the landscape, and then noiselessly moving on. Aching to be with my faithful companion, I could nearly see a robin weep.

That evening I prepared a blazing campfire to keep me warm. Then, using leftover firewood and citronella candles, I created a makeshift shrine. I lit three candles, one for Rosa, one for Joyce, and one for me. In the center I placed a figurine—Little Rosa, smiling calmly like her namesake after wandering with me in the woods. I sat and gazed, as if to say, "I will not let you go." I heard the silence of a falling star lighting up a purple sky. And as I wondered where she was, I was so lonesome I could cry.

14

Homecoming

WHEN DOGS become companions, they and their people can take on each other's best traits. We learn from our canine companions just as they learn from us. I can summarize in two words what Rosa, Joyce, and I learned together at 315 Benjamin Avenue: love and generosity. The house itself, with its spacious living room, sunlit music room, and ample guest rooms, exuded hospitality. We had many occasions to learn what this meant: frequent visits from out-of-town guests, regular receptions for colleagues in the arts and the academy, extended stays by friends in need, and a daily flow of piano students, both young and old, who waited in the living room to begin their lessons or to be picked up by their parents.

Asked to write a character sketch as a school assignment, one of Joyce's piano students, a ninth-grader, wrote an essay titled "Rosa":

> Rosa . . . has a full life. Her family, Joyce and Lambert, a happy couple, live a good life in a beautiful, big, old-fashioned house in a lovely neighborhood with plenty of trees and sidewalks, bushes and squirrels; ideal for evening walks to the park. After piano lessons, art classes, board meetings and the studio, Joyce and Lambert

> come home to a friendly bark and a wag of the tail from an old friend named Rosa.
>
> Rosa is someone who is contented with what she does . . . She keeps watch over the house and many children who come every day, napping in the sunlight streaming through the open stained glass window in the summer, and listening to the familiar music coming from the old grand. Rosa has had her share of being hugged, kissed, petted, and adored by many children with sticky hands and dirty faces. She knows every inch of her house, and loves all who walk through the door.
>
> To me those old eyes know more than what many think; she understands it all when it comes to children, big or small, even though her bones creak and her tail has a curious wag. She has memorized familiar pieces from Bach and knows 9th grade math problems and science questions, though now she tends to sleep the day away or hang out with the black cat, Ebony. Some child will find her and get to know her soul and the young heart she has open for all.[13]

To have a young heart open for all: that is what Joyce and I learned from Rosa. I am learning still.

I grew up in a community where tender feelings are held close to one's chest. The day I left for college was the first time I heard my father cry. He choked back his tears. Yet he was not a macho man. When our family entered church for Sunday services, Dad held the door open for everyone else who arrived at the same time. Our family waited inside as Dad waited for others. Every time I returned home from university, a magical moment would occur when Dad shyly asked, "Say, Lambert, do you need any socks?" It was his way of expressing affection. But the cultural environment then, and the academic profession I entered later, did not encourage emotional openness. In the masculine world of North America, toughness, not tenderness, is the public norm. Although told to be kind and respectful, boys are taught to compete and make war. The result in my own life has been a constant conflict between public assertion and private affection.

An image from my childhood captures this tension. After the Sunday morning church service, Mom's family would gather at Grandma's house for coffee and conversation. Mom was the second youngest child in a large family that emigrated from the Netherlands in 1920. She had six brothers and one much older sister. I never knew Mom's father, after whom I am named—Grandpa Beuving died before I was born. In photographs he appears to be a stern and upright man. My grandma was a kind and caring soul. She showed this mostly through gestures, for she spoke hardly any English, and we grandchildren did not learn Dutch.

Grandma's house was tiny. A wooden-frame, one-story bungalow, it sat on the corner of a quiet intersection in Ripon, California. Outside were a row of orange trees on one side, an unfenced front yard with a loquat tree, and a vegetable garden and chicken coops in the back. Each room inside was smaller than the hallways in many homes. The house was all that my impoverished grandparents could afford when they immigrated to the United States.

In this tiny house all of us gathered for our Sunday "koffieklets," the aunts and uncles, the nieces and nephews, and little great-grandchildren too. The uncles presided over the living room, where they heatedly debated politics and religion while the women served. The aunts hovered in the kitchen and dining room, minding the children, tending to refreshments, and *sotto voce* sharing their lives. Between these rooms roamed the children, playing and listening to the grown-ups talk. Standing between the uncles and the aunties, one could experience a multilayered dissonance worthy of Charles Ives.

Both sets of voices have struggled to be heard in my life ever since: the harsh and opinionated brass of my uncles, and the velvet and muted reeds of my aunts. For years they pulled in opposite directions and became fully audible only in their separate rooms. The rigorous life of a philosopher and campus leader, where one needed to fight for one's views, seemed disconnected from the life of a friend and companion, where nurturing others came first. Although teaching at the university level required both sides to flourish, the two voices always seemed out of sync.

When Joyce and I lived at the Benjamin house with Rosa, the walls of separation weakened, and the resonance of the two voices began to change. Yet it was only in losing Rosa that I became free to transform their destructive dissonances. To be loving, I learned, I need to let the uncles' harshness fade away. And to be generous, I need to let the aunties' muteness go. Then their constricted voices will be released into a gracious and vigorous openness for all. I will be able do philosophy with a human heart. I will sing my own songs in a creative key.

This movement toward freedom is the greatest gift my life with Rosa has received, a gift discovered, paradoxically, through her death. I have learned to bask in unconditional generosity, even when that means dying to parts of my divided self. I have learned like Rosa to listen to the familiar music, freely at home. Thank you, Sister Rosa. Thank you.

15

Postlude: Elegy

"Do you think you will get another dog?" Friends and colleagues began to ask me a couple of months after Rosa died. Two years later the question still comes up. At first I could only say, "No, not yet." A year later I could reply, "Perhaps." It is hard to explain why I hesitate, why I do not actually look for another dog. My lament is a silent song that only the heart can sing.

Joyce and I were visiting friends in Grand Rapids over the Labor Day weekend in 2006 when I first felt ready, after eighteen months, to consider another adoption. I drove to the Humane Society of Kent County by myself. The parking lot was full. Many people were there on a holiday weekend to receive volunteer training or to adopt animals. I asked to see the dogs.

I visited the puppy kennels first. One bears a plaque to recognize our donation several years earlier to the society's new facility: "To honor our wonderful dog Rosa. Lambert Zuidervaart and Joyce Recker." Two puppies immediately caught my eye, both of them blond Labradors, one of them two months old and the other about three. I asked about them, but neither was up for adoption yet.

Then I walked past the adult dogs. A few looked very lovable, and many were eager to be adopted, but none seemed a suitable successor to Rosa. Unsure what to do, I was repeating the tour when one of the workers approached. She said an eight-week-old female puppy had just returned. Adopted a few days earlier, the puppy came back because the adopting family's adult dog had not welcomed her. Did I want to see it? "Sure," I said, "why not?" First I needed to fill out adoption papers and to confirm that it would be ok to transport the puppy to Canada. Then I went through an adoption interview.

After the worker interviewed me, she went out to get the puppy. As she left the interviewing room, she said the puppy was sick with kennel cough. This is not going to work, I immediately thought. How can we travel back to Toronto with a sick puppy and then ask someone else to take care of her the next day, when both Joyce and I will be away? But the worker was already out the door, so I simply waited.

She returned with a sweet, gangly-legged black Lab mix named Petunia. I held Petunia on my lap and pet her. She began to cough deeply. I sat with her a little longer. I whispered to Petunia that she would make someone a good pet. She looked up at me as I talked. Then I told the worker it would be too complicated to travel six or seven hours with a sick puppy. As I said this, Petunia lifted her little head and licked my beard. Fighting my tears, I handed her back, thanked the worker for letting me see her, and said it had been good to visit the kennels. I left quickly, and I wept.

From the Humane Society I drove to Aman Park, where Rosa and I had enjoyed many happy hikes. A stream meanders through the park. Each of several trails winds through dense woods along and away from this stream. Sitting at an isolated bend in the stream where Rosa and

I had often sat, I realized that something profound was at work. I was not ready to adopt another dog. My lament was asking for more time. It could not take a straight path to resolution. It wanted to find images and words beyond the still spaces in my heart. I needed to write this book.

The next day Joyce and our friends and I went for a hike at Hoffmaster State Park. Where the trail turns toward Lake Michigan, Joyce and I parted company from the others. We took a side trail to the spot where I had buried Rosa's dog tag in April 2005. We put our Little Rosa figurine on the grass nearby and sat quietly. Joyce reminded me of my ditty for Rosa. I sang a verse, until tears stopped my song: "Oh, Rosa is a very fine dog, Yes, we love our Rosa . . ." Together we hummed another tune, and Joyce hummed one alone. I told Joyce that my sadness came mixed with gladness, gladness for all the good Rosa had brought into my life.

Some will say such a strong attachment to one companion animal is perverse. They will say it signals a corrupt society where extreme affluence permits unending self-indulgence while human friendship breaks down. As a social philosopher, I recognize these worries and feel their point. Yet I have come to understand that sorrow, like friendship, takes many forms, and that living through our grief is a path to renewal. Companion animals are gifts to receive with thanks. Like all good gifts received aright, they help us become better people. Losing them is no less painful than losing one's closest human friend. It would be perverse not to acknowledge their absence. There is indeed a time to weep.

One day our mourning will turn into dancing. But we do not mourn in order to dance. We mourn in order to give voice to loss and longing too deep for words. When one day a new dog comes prancing into my life, I will love her. I will love her, as I love Rosa, with a love too deep for words, a love in which echoes, like the sound of distant barking, a lilting song of Benjamin.

Acknowledgments

FRIENDSHIP IS a gift to be sung. Although this book tells of a canine companion, it also celebrates human friendships. I would not have so enjoyed Rosa's companionship, nor written about her life and death, if I were not connected to human friends through her. I want to thank them here.

Joyce Recker and I have been married for thirty-three years. We have shared wonderful friendships and grieved significant losses together. Joyce recognized my need to adopt a dog in 1990. She enjoyed Rosa's companionship as much as I did. After Rosa died, Joyce held me close, letting me take time to grieve and upholding my first faltering efforts to find the right words. Joyce, you are a precious gift. Thank you for gracing my life.

My mother, Tena Beuving Zuidervaart, suffered a stroke in August 2007. Our monthly correspondence of nearly forty years ended soon afterwards, and she died in June 2009 at the age of ninety-five. Mom never read *Dog-Kissed Tears*. But her life-long encouragement of my intellectual pursuits lies behind this book. I dedicate it to her memory and to the memory of my father, Martin Zuidervaart, whose presence in the book will be obvious to all who have read it. They, too, have graced my life.

My brother, Martin Zuidervaart, and my sister, Roelyn Poot, read a draft of the book and gave me heartfelt responses. Marty wrote out detailed and insightful comments on the entire manuscript. Roelyn made verbal comments that were equally helpful. Marty and Roelyn gave their blessing to stories that reveal parts of our family's life. I am most grateful.

Ron Otten shared many of Rosa's adventures with me. He lived with Joyce and me for several months when Rosa was one year old, and he accompanied us on camping trips and at family gatherings during the 1990s. Ron helped me to delight in doglike antics and to treasure Rosa's friendship. The e-mail I quote in chapter 10 is a small example of the love and wisdom he has shared. Thank you, Brother Ron. Thank you.

Writing this book required time for reflection and space for solitude that a busy academic life made hard to find. Our friends Connie Bellows and Darlene Zwart opened their house to me for a ten-day writing retreat when they were touring Italy in May 2007. Sitting on their deck by an animated marsh, listening to familiar music in the quiet of their home, and revisiting the West Michigan trails where Rosa and I had hiked, I enjoyed an inspiring place to complete my writing. Thank you, Sisters Connie and Darlene, for your support.

Ron, Connie, and Darlene were among the first to read the manuscript I finished in May 2007. I also shared it with Linda Ruiter, Toni Perrine, and Daryl Fischer. Linda was our housemate in Edmonton during the early 1980s, as was Ron, and she first met Rosa during a 1990 household reunion in Grand Rapids. Joyce and I became friends with Toni when her children took piano lessons from Joyce in the 1990s. Toni often visited us in Toronto during Rosa's last years. I know Daryl from our time together on the Board of the Urban Institute for Contemporary Arts when we helped turn an abandoned commercial building into a contemporary arts center. Linda, Toni, and Daryl understood the importance of my undertaking a much more personal project of creative reconstruction, and they encouraged its completion as a book.

Three other friends with ties to the world of publishing provided seasoned readings and timely advice. Jean Blomquist, my friend since our high school years in California, offered very helpful comments on both the manuscript and a book proposal, drawing from her own experience as a writer and editor. Graeme Burk, the former communications director at the Institute for Christian Studies, the graduate school where I teach, gave me a lively sense of the book's potential audience and urged me to seek publication. Peter Enneson, my former classmate in graduate school and an art director and graphic designer, assured me that the manuscript was publishable and helped me connect with people who could get it published. To all of these friends—Linda, Toni, Daryl, Jean, Graeme, and Peter—I express deep gratitude.

Several of my current and former graduate students, all of them gifted writers, read the manuscript and encouraged its publication: Allyson Carr, Wendy Falb, Matt Klaassen, Janet Read, and Ronnie Shuker. I greatly appreciate their interest in the nonacademic side of my life. I also thank Simona Goi, my former faculty colleague at Calvin College, and Leah (Vanderhill) Schoonover, Joyce's former piano student, for letting me quote their reflections on Rosa.

Music is an important part of my life. I studied piano and French horn growing up, graduated from college with a double major in music and philosophy, and stayed active as a musician and music teacher during my graduate studies in philosophy. After I left graduate school, academic work absorbed ever more energy, and my music making declined. I returned to music when Rosa died, especially to singing. Three people in particular have inspired this return: fellow choir members Karen Johnston and Karen Watson and my vocal instructor, Mervin Fick. My return to music making released imaginative impulses that long had lain dormant. They found articulation in this book. Thank you, Karen, Karen, and Mervin, for helping me sing through my sorrow.

The experiences I sing in this book are intensely personal. I can share them with others thanks to professional help from two gifted counselors. In 1994, as I struggled with losing my father in 1989, I sought spiritual direction from Sister Carmelita Murphy, OP. She was prioress of the Grand Rapids Dominicans at the time. Sister Carmelita had a wonderful ability to listen past my words for the pain they expressed. I learned from her to speak with Dad, five years after his death, about my feelings of loss and my need to know him better. I thank Sister Carmelita for helping me find a voice that for so long seemed lacking.

A decade later I underwent traumatic loss of a different sort and sought help from a psychotherapist. Every week for more than a year Dr. Catherine Carmichael listened attentively to the troubled soul within my verbal associations. As she helped me discover connections beyond the surface of my conscious life, I became acutely aware of suppressed creativity left untended for far too long. I was submerged in this process of self-discovery when Rosa died. Catherine supported me during the difficult months that followed, and she held open a door to personal transformation. Without her professional assistance I could not have considered writing this book. Thank you, Catherine, for helping me gather my tears. Thank you for helping me learn to sing again.

Grieving the loss of a friend takes time. More than two years passed between Rosa's death in February 2005 and my completing the first draft of this book in May 2007. A few months later I finally decided to adopt another dog. It was not an easy decision, and I would not have reached it on my own. Esther Hart, our goddaughter, died of cancer in April 2007. Losing her weighed heavily on Joyce and me. A naturopath I was seeing about physical ailments immediately diagnosed my condition as symptomatic of unresolved grief. She let me know this during my last session with her on July 20, 2007. "Lambert," she declared, "the single most important step you can take along the path of healing is to adopt a puppy—not a dog, but a puppy." Instantly I recognized the truth of her advice. The next day I went online to find a suitable breeder, and the very next morning Joyce and I drove through the Ontario countryside to Cooperslane Kennel to meet the sire and dam of a dozen puppies born on July 7. At the end of August we adopted an eight-week-old purebred Golden Retriever and named her Hannah Estelle.

Rosa Luxemburg Parks will always hold a special place in my heart. Yet there is room, I learned, for a new companion. Like Rosa, Hannah brings smiles and laughter and pleasant times. She loves to invite every visitor to our festival of friends. We will celebrate Hannah's third birthday at Awenda Provincial Park in July. But her story awaits another time.

Lambert Zuidervaart
Toronto
May 24, 2010

Notes

[1] Verses 1 and 2 of Bruce Cockburn, "Festival of Friends," *In the Falling Dark*, True North, 1976.

[2] Verses 1 and 3, with refrain, from "Precious Lord, Take My Hand." Thomas Dorsey wrote the text in 1932 and adapted the music from the tune "Maitland" by George N. Allen (1844).

[3] In its final form, the book contains fifteen chapters arranged in an arch structure, a familiar pattern in cantatas by Johann Sebastian Bach. In an arch structure, each step toward the capstone has its counterpart in a step away. So the first chapter in this book corresponds to the last, the second to the second last, etc., as follows: 1–15, 2–14, 3–13, 4–12, 5–11, 6–10, and 7–9. Resting at the center, chapter 8 divides into two parts, mirroring both sides of the arch and imitating the double chorus from Bach that it quotes.

Thematically the structure is an inverted arch. It descends through the first seven chapters to Rosa's death, and then it ascends beyond her death through the final seven. After an introduction in chapter 1, chapters 2–7 take us through Rosa's first six years. Chapters 9–14 trace my responses to her death in the days and months that follow, until we reach an elegiac coda in chapter 15. This is not a rigid structure, however. Individual chapters move freely between the earlier and later years of Rosa's life, and I wrote them in a different order from their published sequence.

Many chapters feature words from songs whose meaning became even more poignant after Rosa died. These songs are of various sorts and sources: traditional hymns from my childhood, liturgical songs from my adult years, favorite arias and choruses from the classical vocal repertoire, rock songs from the past several decades, and even a homemade ditty sung only to Rosa. I have chosen them for their resonance with the experiences I share, a resonance created as much by the melodies and musical settings as by the lyrics and texts.

[4] From Sting, "Fragile," ...*Nothing Like the Sun*, A&M Records, 1987.

[5] Verses 1 and 4 from "In the Bleak Midwinter," as printed in *Voices United* (Etobicoke, ON: United Church Publishing House, 1996), song no. 55. Christina Rossetti wrote the words as a Christmas poem for *Scribner's Monthly* magazine in 1872. Later they were set to the tune "Cranham" that Gustav Holst composed in 1906.

[6] The German text of this chorus from Johann Sebastian Bach's *Matthäus Passion* (1729) is by the poet Christian Friedrich Henrici, known as Picander. I have provided my own translation.

[7] "Lascia ch'io pianga," from the opera *Rinaldo* (1711) by Georg Friedrich Händel, with Italian libretto by Giacomo Rossi.

[8] Bruce McLeod, "Held by a God Who Hurts Too," *The United Church Observer* (May 2005), pp. 33–34.

[9] From the last verse of Sting, "Fields of Gold," *Ten Summoner's Tales*, A&M Records, 1993.

[10] From "Healer of Our Every Ill," words and music by Marty Haugen, 1987, as printed in *Voices United* (Etobicoke,

ON: United Church Publishing House, 1996), song no. 619.

[11] From "Blest Be the Tie That Binds," text by John Fawcett (1782) and tune attributed to Johann G. Nägeli (1828), as printed in the *Psalter Hymnal* (Grand Rapids, MI: CRC Publications, 1987, 1988), song no. 315.

[12] Verses 3 and 4 from "I'm So Lonesome I Could Cry," originally written and recorded in 1949 by American country music singer and songwriter Hank Williams Sr., and covered by Canadian alternative country rock band The Cowboy Junkies in *The Trinity Session*. Their LP was recorded live at The Church of the Holy Trinity in Toronto on November 27, 1987, released in early 1988 on Latent Records in Canada, and re-released later that year on RCA Records.

[13] Written by Leah Vanderhill, December 1996.

www.ingramcontent.com/pod-product-compliance
Lightning Source LLC
Chambersburg PA
CBHW070326100426

4274 3CB000 11B/2573